Table of Contents

LEAKY GUT DIET COOKBOOK

FOR BEGINNERS AND DUMMIES

ALLEN GOODHART

Copyright

Disclaimer Notice:

Note that it is important that the following information contained in this book is for educational purposes only. After carrying out enough research work, we present a piece of detailed and accurate information as it relates to the present norm. We got the contents in this book from various sources, and hence, the intending readers are not given a warranty. We advise readers to talk to their licensed doctors before trying out the techniques given within this book.

By consenting to this document, the reader accepts that the author is not responsible for any loss either directly or indirectly that can be incurred as a result of the information contained within this book, and also the omissions, errors, or inadequacies of the reader.

Introduction

In recent years, the term "leaky gut" has gotten a lot of attention. Also referred to as increased permeability, it is a phenomenon in which pores in your gut walls begin to loosen. This makes it much easier for bigger substances to move through the intestinal walls and into your bloodstream, such as bacteria, poisons, as well as undigested food particles.

According to research, increased intestinal permeability has been linked to a number of chronic and autoimmune disorders, such as type 1 diabetes and celiac disease.

It all comes down to replacing grains and inflammatory foods with nutrient-dense, natural alternatives, then gradually reintroducing the foods to see how they affect your health.

This book examines the leaky gut diet and its causes in depth. It also offers a variety of tasty and healthy dishes.

Let's get started!

What Is Leaky Gut Syndrome?

Increased intestinal permeability is said to be the cause of the leaky gut syndrome.

The digestive system is made up of several organs that work together to break down food, absorb nutrients and water, and eliminate waste. To keep potentially hazardous substances out of your body, your intestinal lining works as a barrier between your gut and bloodstream.

The highest percentage of nutrient and water absorption takes place in your intestines. Tight junctions or microscopic gaps in your intestines allow nutrients and water to enter your bloodstream.

Gut permeability refers to how easily chemicals flow through the intestinal walls.

These tight connections can weaken due to certain health disorders, potentially allowing dangerous substances such as bacteria, poisons, and undigested food particles to enter your bloodstream.

According to alternative medicine practitioners, leaky gut causes extensive inflammation and activates an immunological response, resulting in a variety of health conditions known as leaky gut syndrome.

They believe leaky gut causes autoimmune illnesses, migraines, autism, food sensitivities, skin disorders, mental fog, and chronic fatigue, among other things.

However, there is minimal evidence to aid the existence of leaky gut syndrome. As a result, it is not recognized as a medical diagnosis by conventional physicians.

Though increased intestinal permeability exists and is associated with a variety of disorders, it's unclear if it's a symptom or the root cause of chronic disease.

What Causes Leaky Gut?

The precise cause of leaky gut is unknown. On the other hand, increased intestinal permeability is well-known and occurs in conjunction with a number of chronic disorders, including celiac disease and type 1 diabetes.

Zonulin

This protein regulates tight junctions. Higher amounts of this protein have been found in studies to loosen tight junctions and promote intestinal permeability.

Bacteria and gluten are two documented causes of elevated zonulin levels in some people.

Gluten increases intestinal permeability in celiac disease patients, according to research.

However, outcomes from studies in healthy adults and people with non-celiac gluten sensitivity are equivocal.

While gluten has been shown to enhance intestinal permeability in test tubes, no such effect has been reported in human trials.

Other factors, in addition to zonulin, can promote intestinal permeability.

Inflammatory mediators, including tumour necrosis factor (TNF) and interleukin 13 (IL-13), as well as long-term usage of nonsteroidal anti-inflammatory medicines (NSAIDs) like aspirin and ibuprofen, have been shown to enhance intestinal permeability in studies.

Low quantities of beneficial gut flora may also have the same impact. This is referred to as gut dysbiosis.

What To Eat

- Mushrooms

- A variety of vegetables

- Healthy animal fats, olive oil & coconut oil

- Quality meats, preferably pasture-raised and organic

- Fermented foods

- Fruit at moderate levels

- Glycine-rich foods like bone broth

- Spices that aren't derived from seeds

What Not To Eat

- Legumes, including soy and peanuts

- Grains, especially gluten

- Refined sugars

- Dairy

- Eggs

- Industrial seed oils

- Nuts

- Nightshades, including tomatoes, potatoes, sweet, eggplant, and tomatillos, hot peppers, and spices from peppers such as paprika, cayenne peppers, red pepper flakes, etc.

- Seeds and spices derived from seeds (such as nutmeg, coriander seed, mustard seed, etc.)

- Chocolate

- Alcohol

- Sweeteners, including artificial, stevia, and monk fruit

- Nonsteroidal anti-inflammatory drugs such as ibuprofen

- Emulsifiers, thickeners, and other food additives

It may seem difficult to stick to the rules, but it's critical to do so for the first 4 to 6 weeks so that your body doesn't continue to produce antibodies to any dietary proteins that could be triggering. When it comes to reintroduction foods, you can start with those that are least likely to trigger responses or with the ones that may have the most benefits from being taken back in, such as eggs with their nutrient-dense yolks. Working with a dietitian, nutritionist, or health coach to guide you through the reintroduction process might be beneficial.

How Is AIP Related to Leaky Gut?

Although the medical diagnosis of leaky gut is still debated, the concept of intestinal permeability has been reported in medical literature for over a century.

Intestinal permeability has been associated with celiac disease, irritable bowel syndrome (IBS), and Crohn's disease in studies.

Doctors are now attempting to determine how common the consequences of a leaky gut are. Some experts believe there isn't enough evidence to link particular symptoms to hyperpermeability, while others believe the leaky gut syndrome is one of the leading crises of our time, affecting an estimated 50 million individuals.

Doctors are now investigating these distinctions.

The AIP diet tries to eliminate inflammatory foods and replace them with nutrient-dense, easy-to-digest foods. This should help repair your intestines by closing up the "holes" over time.

The goal of this "healing" is to:

- Reduce the signs and symptoms of Autoimmune Disease

- Reducing autoimmune reactions

- Regain control of your immune system

- Prevent the occurrence of secondary autoimmune disorders.

A One-Day Leaky Gut Diet Meal Plan.

Try this sample menu to get started on a leaky gut diet, but feel free to mix and match or substitute foods from the list above:

Breakfast: Two scrambled eggs with sautéed kale on the side. (Helpful hint: When starting a leaky gut diet, cooked veggies are easier on the gut and may be a better choice than raw). Do you crave something sweet? A bowl of oats with almond milk, berries, and walnuts is a delicious option.

Lunch: A salad with lentils & lean protein will give you long-lasting energy and a healthy dose of prebiotic fibre. Probiotics can be added in the form of kimchi or sauerkraut. Salads aren't your cup of tea? Fill romaine lettuce with tuna or chicken salad (prepared with an avocado-oil-based mayo) and eat it like a taco!

Snack: Carrot slices with hummus, apple slices with almond butter, or crisp roasted chickpeas are good options for a snack. The options are unlimited, but leaky-gut snacks should include some gut-friendly fibre, as well as a little amount of fat and protein to help maintain blood sugar stability.

Dinner: Consider the following formula: high-quality protein source + non-starchy veggie + starchy veggie (optional) + healthy fat. Salmon pan-seared with roasted sweet potato & Brussels sprouts cooked in olive oil would be ideal. Is there another option? Noodles made with zucchini, pesto, sun-dried tomatoes & grilled chicken.

Other Ways To Improve Your Gut Health

Although eating is essential for gut health, there are many other things you can do. Here are a few more things you can do to help your gut health:

Taking A Probiotic Supplement Is A Good Idea.

Beneficial bacteria found naturally in fermented foods are found in probiotics. If you don't receive enough probiotics from your diet, taking a probiotic supplement, which you can get online, may help.

Reduce Your Stress Levels.

It has been proven that chronic stress harms healthy gut microorganisms. Meditation and yoga, for example, can be beneficial.

Smoking Should Be Avoided.

Cigarette smoking has been linked to a number of bowel diseases and has been shown to cause inflammation in the digestive tract. Quitting smoking can increase the number of beneficial bacteria in your gut while decreasing the number of dangerous bacteria.

More Sleep Is Required.

Sleep deprivation can influence an imbalance in the distribution of beneficial bacteria in the gut, perhaps leading to increased intestinal permeability.

Limit Your Alcohol Consumption.

According to research, excessive alcohol use has been demonstrated to enhance intestinal permeability by interacting with specific proteins.

Consider being tested for celiac disease if you suspect you have the leaky gut syndrome. Symptoms of the two illnesses may be similar. Diets like the Gut and Psychology Syndrome (GAPS) diet have also been shown to help persons with leaky gut symptoms. This diet, however, is extremely restrictive, and there are no scientific studies to back up its health claims.

AIP Avocado Coconut Smoothie

Preparation Time: 5 Minutes

Cook Time: 0 Minutes

Yields: 2 Servings

Recipes

- One cup of ice

- One ripe avocado

- One teaspoon of raw honey, to taste

- ½ cup of unsweetened coconut milk – add a little bit more if desired

Directions

1. Cut the avocado in half.

2. Next, use a spoon to scoop out the flesh of the avocado.

3. Place the avocado flesh into a clean blender with the coconut milk, raw honey and ice, and then blend well (gradually increase the speed).

4. Add more coconut milk if required to blend until smooth.

AIP Green Detox Juice

Preparation Time: 10 Minutes

Cook Time: 10 Minutes

Yields: 1 Serving

Recipes:

- One small Granny Smith apple, core removed & roughly chopped
- 5.3 ounces of kale, roughly chopped
- One lemon, rind & pips removed and diced
- 3.5 ounces or about 5 stalks of celery, roughly chopped
- One thumb-size piece ginger, peeled and roughly diced
- Handful mint leaves

Directions

1. Place all the recipes into a clean juicer and switch on the juicer.

2. As soon as it is done, discard the pulp. Stir the juice well and enjoy with ice, if desired.

Carrot Apple Banana Smoothie

Preparation Time: 10 Minutes

Cook Time: 0 minutes

Yields: 1 Serving

Recipes:

- Half carrot (about 3 ounces), chopped

- One apple, chopped

- One cup of ice

- One banana

- Half tablespoon of coconut oil

- Dash of cinnamon

- Half cup of coconut milk

Directions

Add all the recipes into a clean blender and blend well until smooth.

Avocado Green Smoothie

Preparation Time: 5 Minutes

Cook Time: 0 Minutes

Yields: 1 Serving

Recipes:

- One ripe banana

- Half ripe avocado

- Half cup of coconut milk (or water)

- One cup of ice

- One handful of greens of your choice (spinach, kale, chard)

Directions

1. Place the banana, avocado and ice into the clean blender.

2. Top with your desired greens.

3. Now blend until it is smooth (add additional coconut milk or water if you have difficult blending it).

Blueberry Mint Smoothie

Preparation Time: 10 Minutes

Cook Time: 0 Minutes

Yields: 1 Servings

Recipes:

- Half cup of coconut milk (or water)

- Half cup of frozen blueberries

- Half avocado

- 3/4 cup of ice (about 4 large ice cubes made from this ice cube tray)

- One teaspoon of mint tea leaves (or about 10 fresh mint leaves)

Directions

1. Gently pour the coconut milk into a clean blender.

2. Add frozen blueberries, avocado (use a spoon to scoop out the flesh), ice cubes, mint leaves and then blend until smooth.

Easy Pumpkin Smoothie

Preparation Time: 5 Minutes

Total Time: 6 Minutes

Yields: 1 Serving

Recipes:

- Half cup of pumpkin purée

- 3/4 cup of coconut milk

- Three tablespoons of collagen protein or vegan protein powder

- 1/4 of an avocado

- One tablespoon of maple syrup (or sugar-free sweetener)

- One teaspoon of cinnamon

- One tablespoon of coconut butter

- Half teaspoon of vanilla extract

- One tablespoon of coconut oil

- One cup ice cubes (optional)

- One drop Thieves essential oil (optional)

Directions

Combine all recipes in a clean blender and blend. Add ice cubes or water to attain desired consistency.

AIP Red Velvet Smoothie

Preparation Time: 10 Minutes

Cook Time: 0 minutes

Yields: 1 Serving

Recipes:

- One banana, peeled & diced

- One large beet, cooked, peeled & diced

- Half cup of full-fat coconut milk

- One tablespoon of carob powder

- One tablespoon of coconut cream, to drizzle (optional)

- Half cup of crushed ice

Directions

Place the beets, banana, coconut milk & crushed ice into a blender & blitz until it is fairly smooth.

Now pour into a glass and drizzle over a little whisked coconut cream before enjoying!

AIP Tropical Smoothie

Preparation Time: 5 Minutes

Cook Time: 0 Minutes

Yields: 2 Servings

Recipes:

- 6 ounces of coconut water

- One banana, peeled and diced

- Three tablespoons of full-fat coconut milk

- 14 ounces of pineapple chunks

Directions

1. Place the recipes in a clean blender and then combine until entirely smooth.

2. Transfer the smoothie into two chilled glasses and then serve to enjoy.

AIP Strawberry Banana Smoothie

Prep Time: 5 minutes

Cook Time: 0 Minutes

Yields: 1 Serving

Recipes:

- One ripe banana
- 8 strawberries
- One teaspoon of MCT oil
- One cup of ice
- Half cup of coconut milk

Directions

Place all the recipes into a clean blender and then blend.

Egg-Free Paleo Macaroons

Serves: 12 macaroons

Recipes:

- 1 tablespoon of coconut flour

- 1½ cups of unsweetened shredded coconut

- 2 tablespoons of coconut oil, melted

- ⅛ teaspoon of celtic sea salt

- 1 tablespoon of vanilla extract

- ¼ cup of honey

Directions

1. Combine coconut flour & shredded coconut in a clean food processor.

2. Pulse in coconut oil, salt, vanilla and honey.

3. Gently scoop batter one level tablespoon at a time onto a parchment paper lined baking sheet

4. Bake at 350 degrees Fahrenheit for seven to ten minutes.

5. Cool for one hour

6. Serve to enjoy.

Paleo Pumpkin Chili (Nightshade-Free)

Recipes:

- Half onion, chopped

- One teaspoon of olive oil

- Two to three cloves garlic, chopped

- Two cups of beef broth

- One-pound ground grass-fed beef or ground turkey

- Half can pumpkin purée

- Two cups of butternut squash, cubed

- Half teaspoon of apple cider vinegar

- One beet, cooked and puréed

- One teaspoon of oregano

- One teaspoon of cinnamon

- 1/4 teaspoon of turmeric

- 1/4 teaspoon of ground cloves

- One bay leaf

- Half teaspoon of salt

Directions

1. Fisrtly, heat the olive oil in a large clean Dutch oven over medium to high heat. Add the onion & garlic and sauté until it gets tender.

2. Now add the ground meat, breaking up using a clean spoon. Cook until it turns brown.

3. Next deglaze the pan with beef broth, scraping the sides and bottom. Add the bay leaf and spices.

4. Next reduce the heat to low and then add pumpkin purée, the butternut squash, apple cider vinegar and beet purée. Stir until well it is combined.

5. Now cover and then simmer for twenty to thirty minutes, until the butternut squash gets tender.

6. Go ahead to serve with your desired toppings!

Simple AIP Dessert With Plantains And Raspberries

Recipes:

- Raspberries and coconut milk to serve

- Organic coconut oil to fry

- Ripe plantain

Directions

Carefully slice a ripe plantain and then fry in an organic coconut oil until it is just crispy on all sides. Serve with some raspberries ad a drizzle of coconut milk.

"Curried" Chicken Salad

Recipes:

- Half avocado

- Six ounces cooked shredded chicken

- One chopped scallion

- Two tablespoons of full-fat coconut cream

- A few shakes of turmeric and cinnamon

- Two tablespoons chopped cilantro

- A squeeze of lime juice

- Lots of salt

Directions

1. Chop or shred chicken into bite-sized pieces.

2. In a clean container, combine coconut cream, avocado, cilantro, green onion, lime juice and spices. Mash using a clean fork until it is creamy.

3. Add the chicken and mix until squarely coated. Season to with salt to your taste.

4. Serve with or without lettuce wraps!

AIP Basil Pesto

Recipes:

- Two cloves of garlic, crushed

- Five cups tightly packed fresh organic basil

- One teaspoon of sea salt

- One cup of organic extra virgin olive oil

- One teaspoon of freshly squeezed lemon juice

Directions

1. Rinse the basil and remove the leaves.

2. Add the basil leaves and the remaining recipes to the blender.

3. Blend on medium speed for one minute until it is well combined.

Note

It can be stored in the refrigerator for up to 5 days or frozen to extend the storage life.

AIP Chicken And Tarragon Breakfast Sausages

Preparation Time: 5 Minutes

Cook Time: 15 Minutes

Yields: 4 Servings

Recipes:

- Two tablespoons of tarragon, finely chopped (or other preferred herbs)

- One pound of ground chicken

- Four tablespoons of coconut oil, for cooking

- One teaspoon of salt

Directions

1. Add the ground chicken, salt, and finely chopped tarragon in a clean container. Using your hands, split the mixture into eight equal amounts and shape each part into a firm, flat sausage patty.

2. Now heat the coconut oil in a clean pan and then gently fry the sausages over medium heat on all sides for ten to fifteen minutes. Using a meat thermometer monitor the internal temperature till it reaches 165 degrees Fahrenheit.

AIP Ground Beef Stroganoff with Spinach

Preparation Time: 5 Minutes

Cook Time: 30 Minutes

Calories: 651kcal

Yields: 4 Servings

Recipes:

- One tablespoon of Extra Virgin Olive Oil

- One Onion chopped

- Two teaspoons of Salt

- One pound Ground Beef

- One and a half teaspoon of Dried Thyme

- Two teaspoons of Garlic Powder

- One teaspoon of Cinnamon

- Half cup of Coconut Cream optional

- One and a half teaspoon of Ground Ginger

- One cup of Bone Broth

- One pinch of Ground Cloves

- Five ounces of Baby Spinach

- Eight ounces of Sweet Potato Noodles

Directions

1. Firstly, bring a stock pot of water to a boil.

2. Next add onions to a large clean sauté pan with olive oil over medium to high heat until onions gets translucent.

3. Next add the ground beef and then break apart with a clean spoon.

4. Next add the spices and herbs then stir to combine.

5. Next pour the broth over the meat mixture and then bring to a boil on high heat.

6. Allow the beef mixture cook for around ten minutes, occasionally stirring.

7. As the beef is cooking, add the sweet potato starch noodles to the stockpot and then cook for around six to eight minutes.

8. As soon as the noodles are finished cooking, add the noodles to the pan of ground beef.

9. Now add the spinach to the noodles and then toss to combine.

10. Add cream to the pan if you are using any and then toss another time. Ensure to coat the noodles evenly with the sauce.

11. Serve to enjoy.

Garlic and Thyme Chicken Meal

Prep

Preparation Time: 15 Minutes

Cook Time: 20 Minutes

Total Time: 35 Minutes

Calories: 326kcal

Yields: 3 Servings

Recipes:

- Five cups of Brussels Sprouts, rinsed, trim and halved

- Three 4 ounces of Chicken Breasts

- Three cloves of garlic

- Two tablespoons of olive oil

- One large sweet potato, rinsed and chopped into half-inch cubes

- Two tablespoons of dried thyme

- Fresh thyme

- One teaspoon of Salt

Directions

1. Oven to 425 degrees Fahrenheit

2. Next place the chicken breast in a zip lock bag with dried thyme, two tablespoons of olive oil, half teaspoon of salt and garlic. Zip the bag and rub the spices and oil into the chicken.

3. Place the brussels sprouts in large clean bowl, add one tablespoon of olive oil, add the sweet potato. Microwave for three minutes to soften. Toss in one tablespoon of the olive oil.

4. Next place the brussels and sweet potatoes on a sheet pan lined with parchment paper or tin foil. Sprinkle with half teaspoon of salt. Take out chicken from bag and then place on the sheet pan.

5. Next bake for twenty to twenty-five minutes or until chicken is well cooked through.

6. Last garnish with fresh thyme to enjoy.

AIP Ground Beef Breakfast Casserole

Preparation Time: 20 Minutes

Cook Time: 35 Minutes

Yields: 8 Servings

Recipes:

- Three tablespoons of avocado oil, to cook the ground beef and onions with

- 1.5 pounds of ground beef

- One cup of coconut cream (from the tops of 2 refrigerated cans of coconut milk)

- One medium onion, diced

- Two peaches (or apples), diced small

- Half head of cauliflower, broken into florets

- Two tablespoons of lemon juice

- Four cups of spinach, chopped

- Salt, to taste

- Two tablespoons of fresh parsley, chopped

Directions

1. Oven to 400 degrees Fahrenheit.

2. Grease a large clean casserole baking dish with the one tablespoon of the avocado oil and put aside.

3. Add the three tablespoons of avocado oil to a large clean frying pan and brown the onions and beef. Season with some salt.

4. In a clean blender, blend the cauliflower florets with the coconut cream.

5. Mix the onions, beef and the recipes left in a large clean container. Season with some salt. Pour the mixture into the baking dish (greased).

6. Now bake for thirty-five minutes.

AIP Guacamole Sweet Potato Toast

Preparation Time: 10 Minutes

Cook Time: 30 Minutes

Yields: 4 Servings

Recipes:

- Two tablespoons of avocado oil
- Two small sweet potatoes, ends removed and sliced lengthwise into ¼-inch thick slices
- Salt

For the Guacamole:

- Two tablespoons of garlic powder
- Two large avocados, mashed

- One tablespoon of lime juice

- One tablespoon of onion powder

- Salt

- Two tablespoons of fresh cilantro, finely chopped

Directions

1. Oven to 400 degrees Fahrenheit.

2. On a lightly greased rimmed baking sheet place sweet potato slices.

3. On each of the slices, rub avocado oil and salt. Move all to the baking sheet and then bake for fifteen minutes.

4. Gently turn over each slice and keep on baking for an extra fifteen minutes.

For the Guacamole:

1. In a clean container, combine the garlic powder, avocados, onion powder, fresh cilantro and lime juice. Season with salt, to taste.

2. Top the toasted sweet potato with guacamole, serve to enjoy.

AIP Chicken Breakfast Casserole

Preparation Time: 10 Minutes

Cook Time: 35 Minutes

Yields: 6 Servings

Recipes:

- Three tablespoons of avocado oil, to cook the chicken and onions with

- One tablespoon of avocado oil, to grease baking dish

- One medium onion, thinly sliced

- Two chicken breasts, diced

- One cup of coconut cream (from the tops of two refrigerated cans of coconut milk)

- Half head of cauliflower, chopped

- Four cups of spinach, chopped

- Two tablespoons of lemon juice

- Two carrots, thinly sliced

- Salt, to taste

- Two tablespoons of fresh parsley, chopped

Directions

1. Oven to 400 degrees Fahrenheit.

2. Now grease a large casserole baking dish with the one tablespoon of avocado oil and put aside.

3. Add the three tablespoons of avocado oil to a large clean frying pan and brown the sliced onions and chicken.

4. Mix the onions, chicken, and the recipes left in a large clean container. Season with salt. Transfer mixture into the baking dish (greased).

5. Now bake for thirty-five minutes until the chicken is well cooked and the vegetables gets tender.

Vegan Cheese Sauce

Preparation Time: 20 Minutes

Cook Time: 5 Minutes

Total Time: 10 Hours 25 Minutes

Calories: 115kcal

Yields: 4 Servings

Recipes:

- Half cup of sweet potato, steamed

- Half cup of coconut cream, (add more cream to your thickness preferences)

- 1/4 teaspoon of sea salt

- One teaspoon of nutritional yeast flakes

Directions

1. Begin by steaming the sweet potatoes. Ensure it is fully cooked, but shouldn't be mushy. I used a stovetop using a steamer basket, but you can as well put a little water into a large clean microwave safe bowl/container, add the chopped sweet potato and then microwave in thirty second increments until it gets softened.

2. Shak before opening the can of the coconut cream to combine the cream well with any coconut water present in the can.

3. Pour half a cup into a clean blender, add the remaining half cup of sweet potato, sea salt and nutritional yeast.

4. Now blend to combine the mix.

5. Proceed to heat the sauce entirely over the stovetop or covered in a microwave safe dish/bowl/container.

6. Serve to enjoy.

Paleo Pizza

Preparation Time: 20 Minutes

Cook Time: 30 Minutes

Total Time: 50 Minutes

Calories: 260 kcal

Yields: 8 Servings

Recipes:

For the Crust:

- Two tablespoons of grass-fed gelatin

- 3/4 cup of purified water boiling

- Half cup of coconut flour

- One and a half cups of tapioca flour

- Half teaspoon of baking soda

- Half teaspoon of sea salt

- One teaspoon of apple cider vinegar

- Half cup of sustainable palm shortening room temperature (sub coconut oil)

For the Nightshade-Free "No-Mato" Sauce:

- Four medium carrots, peeled and shredded

- Four large beets, peeled and shredded

- Two teaspoons of garlic minced

- Four cups of beef broth

- Half cup of fresh basil chopped, for garnish

- Half teaspoon of black pepper

For the Toppings:

- Asparagus chopped

- Grass-fed ground beef sauteed

- Herbs

- Leafy greens

Note:

(Use any combination of meat & vegetables that you desire)

Directions

For the Crust:

1. Oven to 400 degrees Fahrenehit. Gently line a baking sheet using clean parchment paper.

2. Next combine the gelatin and hot water in a clean small, heatproof bowl/container. Stir until the gelatin is melted. Put aside.

3. In a different bowl/container, mix together the coconut flour, tapioca, baking soda and salt.

4. Now add the fat to the flour mixture and mix combine well. Add the gelatin water and vinegar to the flour mixture and stir well to combine.

5. Place the dough on the clean lined baking sheet and form into a circle, about 1/4 to 1/3 inch thick.

6. Now bake the crust for fifteen minutes and take out of the oven. Add your desired toppings and bake for additional fifteen minutes, until appears golden brown.

For the No-Mato Sauce:

1. Place all other recipes except the basil in a large clean saucepan and then bring to a simmer over medium heat. Ensure it is covered and simmer for thirty minutes, or until the vegetables gets ender.

2. With an immersion blender to puree the mixture. If the sauce looks too thin, simmer for an additional five to ten minutes, leave uncovered.

3. Modify seasonings to taste.

4. Enjoy!

AIP Ground Beef Stroganoff with Spinach

Preparation Time: 5 Minutes

Cook Time: 30 Minutes

Calories: 651kcal

Yields: 4 Servings

Recipes:

- One tablespoon of Extra Virgin Olive Oil

- One onion, chopped

- Two teaspoons of Salt

- One pound of Ground Beef

- One and a half teaspoon of Dried Thyme

- Two teaspoons of Garlic Powder

- One teaspoon of Cinnamon

- One and a half teaspoon of Ground Ginger

- One cup of Bone Broth

- A pinch Ground Cloves

- Eight ounces of Sweet Potato Noodles

- Half cup of Coconut Cream optional

- Five ounces of Baby Spinach

Directions

1. Firstly, bring a clean stock pot of water to a boil.

2. Add onions to a large clean sauté pan with olive oil over high heat until onions appear translucent.

3. Add the ground beef and then with a clean spoon, break apart.

4. Add in the spices and herbs then stir to combine well.

5. Carefully pour the broth over the meat mixture and then bring to a boil over high heat.

6. Allow the beef mixture to cook for approximately ten minutes, occasionally stirring.

7. Just as the beef is cooking, add the sweet potato starch noodles to the stockpot and cook for approximately six to eight minutes.

8. As soon as the noodles are finished cooking, transfer them to the pan of ground beef

9. Add the spinach to the noodles and then toss to combine well.

10. Add cream to the pan and then toss again, if you are using. Ensure the noodles well coated with the sauce.

11. Serve to enjoy.

Creamy Cauliflower Noodles with Citrus Basil Sauce

Preparation Time: 5 Minutes

Cook Time: 45 Minutes

Total Time: 50 Minutes

Yields: 8 Servings

Recipes:

For the Cauliflower:

- Two tablespoons of avocado oil

- One large head of cauliflower, cut into small florets

- One teaspoon of granulated garlic

- One teaspoon of sea salt

For the Sauce:

- Three cloves of garlic

- One bunch of fresh basil, around three cups (purple, Thai or regular)

- One cup of avocado oil

- One cup of pre-soaked, and drained cashews

- Two teaspoons of fish sauce

- One tablespoon of lemon zest

- Half teaspoon of fine salt

For the Noodles:

- Two packs Miracle Noodle or your desired veggie noodles

Directions

1. Oven to 400 degrees Fahrenheit.

2. Gently toss the cauliflower florets with garlic, oil and salt. Spread out in a large clean casserole dish.

Roast for thirty-five minutes or until appears golden.

3. While it roasts blend all of the sauce recipes in a clean blender untilit is smooth. Put aside.

For the Noodles:

1. Shirataki noodle packets, drain them, and place the noodles in a large clean bowl/container. Cover with some fresh water and soak for five minutes then rinse and drain.

2. As soon as the cauliflower appears golden, open the oven, take out the casserole dish, add the noodles and all of the sauce. Mix all using tongs then spread out evenly in the clean casserole dish.

3. Place back to the oven and bake for fifteen minutes. Take out of the oven and then serve to enjoy!

Broiled Salmon

Preparation Time: 20 Minutes

Cook Time: 8 Minutes

Total Time: 28 Minutes

Yields: 6 Servings

Recipes:

- One teaspoon of fine salt

- 1 1/2 pounds of Side of wild caught salmon

- 1/4 cup of coconut aminos

- Two tablespoon of olive oil

- Chives, for garnish

- 1/4 cup of fresh squeezed orange juice

Directions

1. Gently line sheet pan with a clean parchment paper. Put aside.

2. Season the salmon all over with salt.

3. Combine the olive oil, orange juice and coconut aminos in a shallow bowl/container, big enough for the salmon.

4. Place the salmon meat side down in the marinade. Allow it sit for twenty minutes.

5. Oven to broil 550 degrees Fahrenheit.

6. Now gently place the salmon skin side down on the parchment paper. Pour the aminos, olive oil and juice over it.

7. Broil for eight minutes or until is it well cooked or flakes easily using a clean fork. After eight minutes, check every minute until it's done.

8. Take out of the oven, garnish with the chives.

9. Serve hot to enjoy!

Note:

Goes well with The Crispy Fried Rice, Best Roasted Broccoli or Brussel Sprouts.

AIP Tigernut Granola

Preparation Time: 5 Minutes

Cook Time: 7 Minutes

Yield: 4 Servings

Recipes:

- One ounce coconut flakes

- Six ounce tigernuts

- One tablespoon of honey

- Two ounce mixed dried fruit

Directions

1. Oven to 350 degrees Fahrenheit.

2. Combine the coconut flakes, tigernuts, honey and dried fruit together in a container. Stir until it is well coated.

3. Next spread out in an even layer on a large clean roasting tray and then place in the oven for around six to seven minutes. Take out the tray from the oven put aside to cool finally.

4. Store in a clean airtight container.

Coconut Blueberry Paleo

Oatmeal

Recipes:

- Two ripe bananas, broken into pieces medium to large size

- One cup of full fat organic coconut milk

- One pinch sea salt

- 1/4 cup of coconut butter or coconut manna

- One tablespoon of grass-fed gelatin

- 1 1/4 - 1 1/2 cups finely shredded coconut (determines the thickness of the oatmeal)

- One cup of fresh blueberries

Directions

1. Place a clean pot on the stove on medium heat.

2. Add the bananas, coconut milk, coconut butter, sea salt and vanilla extract to the pot.

3. Now bring to a boil.

4. Next reduce the heat and simmer for ten minutes, stirring every few minutes to let the banana pieces break up.

5. Add the gelatin and stir thoroughly to dissolve

6. Now add the blueberries and cook for another two to three minutes

7. Take away from the heat and add the shredded coconut until it you attain your desired thickness.

8. Next let sit for about five minutes to let the coconut to soften

9. Serve!

Braised Chicken and Leeks

Preparation Time: 15 Minutes

Cook Time: 20 Minutes

Total Time: 35 Minutes

Calories: 294kcal

Yields: 4 Servings

Recipes:

- One pound of Boneless and Skinless Chicken Thighs
- Salt
- Five tablespoons of Clarified Butter AIP Reintroduction or lard, divided
- Ground Pepper optional
- Four Cloves of garlic, chopped
- Three Leeks, cleaned and sliced

- One cup of Chicken Broth

- One teaspoon of Dried Thyme

Directions

1. Firstly, melt three tablespoons of butter in a sauté pan over medium heat.

2. Next sprinkle pepper and salt over the chicken thighs and then add to the sauté pan.

3. Next cook for around two to three minutes per side then take out the chicken from the pan and put aside.

4. Next in the same pan, melt the two tablespoons of butter left over medium heat.

5. Next add the dried thyme, leeks and garlic to the pan and sauté for around three to six minutes or until the leeks are just begins to soften.

6. Next slowly add the chicken broth to the pan and then bring to a boil.

7. Take the chicken back to the pan and then nestle the thighs into the broth and leeks.

8. Turn down the pan to low, cover and then allow to simmer for approximately eight to ten minutes.

9. Put off the heat and serve straightaway.

Chicken Provencal

Preparation Time: 20 Minutes

Cook Time: 1 Hour

Total Time: 1 Hour 20 Minutes

Calories: 349kcal

Yields: 6 Servings

Recipes:

- Salt

- Six to eight Chicken Thighs bone-in, skin-on (about three pounds)

- Half cup of Arrowroot Flour

- Two tablespoons of Herbs de Provence (ensure it's AIP)

- Two tablespoons of Extra Virgin Olive Oil

- Four to six medium-size Shallots, peeled and halved

- Eight to ten Garlic, peeled

- Four sprigs of Thyme or Lavender, for serving

- 1/3 cup of Chicken Broth

Directions

1. Oven to 400 degrees Fahrenheit.

2. Next season the chicken with some salt.

3. Next put the flour in a clean shallow pan, and dredge the chicken in it lightly, shake the pieces to discard excess flour.

4. Next swirl the oil in a large clean roasting pan, and then place the floured chicken in it.

5. Next place the shallots and the garlic around the chicken.

6. Next pour the chicken broth over the top.

7. Now season the chicken with the herbs de Provence.

8. Next put the pan into the oven, and then roast for twenty-five to thirty minutes, then grease it with the pan juices. use an extra two tablespoons of olive oil if there is not enough liquid in the pan.

9. Next keep roasting for an additional twenty-five to thirty minutes, or until the meat cooked through and the chicken skin is very crisp and.

10. Serve in the pan, garnished with the lavender and thyme.

Sweet Potato Chicken Poppers

Preparation Time: 20 Minutes

Cook Time: 40 Minutes

Total Time: 1 Hour

Calories: 62kcal

Yields: 18 Servings

Recipes:

- Two cups of Sweet Potatoes or Yams, about one medium yam, peeled and chopped

- One tablespoon of Extra Virgin Olive Oil

- Three tablespoons of Tapioca Flour

- One pound of Ground Chicken

- Two teaspoons of Garlic Powder

- One teaspoon of Salt

- One teaspoon of Onion Powder

Required Equipment:

- Food Processor or High-Speed Blender

- Large Baking Sheet

Directions

1. Oven to 350 degrees Fahrenheit.

2. Grease a large clean baking sheet with the olive oil over and then put aside.

3. Next add the sweet potatoes to a food processor or high-speed blender then blend until around the size of rice.

4. Next add the sweet potatoes along with the tapioca flour, chicken, garlic powder, salt and onion powder to a large clean mixing bowl/container.

5. With a clean spoon or hands, mix until it is totally combined. To form the poppers, form all into balls

then flatten until each are about one inch thick & in the shape of an egg. Now place the finished poppers on the baking sheet.

6. Next place the entire baking sheet into the oven for forty minutes, flipping midway. As soon as it is finished, take out of the oven and then serve instantly.

AIP Curry Shrimp and Pork Burger

Preparation Time: 30 Minutes

Cook Time: 30 Minutes

Total Time: 1 Hour

Calories: 296kcal

Yields: 6 Servings

Recipes:

- One pound of Ground Pork

- One cup of AIP Thai Yellow Curry Paste (AIP Thai Green Curry Paste is a great alternative)

- One teaspoon of Fish Sauce

- One pound of Shrimp peeled, deveined and then roughly chopped

- Bib Lettuce Leaves used as buns

- One tablespoon of Extra Virgin Olive Oil

Optional Toppings:

- Avocados peeled, pitted and sliced

- Green Onions sliced

- Cilantro leaves

Required Equipment:

- Large Baking Sheet

Directions

1. Oven to 425 degrees Fahrenheit. Add the pork, curry, shrimp and fish sauce in a large clean bowl/container.

2. Next combine then shape into six to eight patties.
   Then cook for thirty minutes.

3. Serve along with lettuce as your bun, avocados,
   green onions and cilantro.

AIP Beef Stew

Preparation Time: 20 Minutes

Cook Time: 3 Hours 30 Minutes

Total Time: 3 Hours 50 Minutes

Calories: 400kcal

Yields: 6 Servings

Recipes:

- Two teaspoons of Salt plus additional for serving

- Two pounds of Stew Beef or Beef Chuck Roast, trimmed and cut into one – one and a half-inch cubes

- Two tablespoons of Ghee AIP reintroduction, substitute with additional olive oil

- Two tablespoons of Extra Virgin Olive Oil

- Three cloves of garlic, minced

- One Onion, diced

- Six cups of Beef Broth Chicken Broth is a good substitute

- One cup of Celery diced

- One tablespoon of Dried Italian Seasoning

- Two tablespoons of Coconut Aminos

- Fresh parsley to garnish (optional)

- Four cups of Root Vegetables peeled and chopped into pieces about half-inch

Required Equipment:

- Stock Pot or Dutch Oven

Directions

1. Firstly, sprinkle two teaspoons of salt over the beef pieces then put aside. Warm olive oil and butter in a

clean heavy bottom stockpot or large dutch oven, over high heat. Then add beef and brown the sides.

2. As soon as all beef is browned, add garlic, celery and onion and then cook until it gets translucent, around five to ten minutes.

3. Next add the Italian seasoning, coconut aminos and beef broth and then stir to combine evenly. Cover and then bring to a boil. When it is boiling, decrease to simmer. Let soup to simmer for two hours thirty minutes.

4. Add carrots and sweet potatoes. Stir to coat the vegetables and then cover. Cook until vegetables are fork tender or for extra thirty minutes.

5. Next taste broth, add extra salt to taste, if required.

6. Garnish with fresh parsley and serve to enjoy.

Notes

1. This recipe calls for parsnips, carrots and sweet potato but any root vegetable will work.

2. Ensure you brown the beef. It helps to make the deep flavourful broth.

3. You can prepare Bone broth with either beef or chicken.

Ginger Mashed Sweet Potatoes

Preparation Time: 20 Minutes

Cook Time: 20 Minutes

Total Time: 40 Minutes

Calories: 310kcal

Yields: 4 Servings

Recipes:

- One cup of Chicken Broth aka Bone Broth

- Two pounds of Sweet Potatoes peeled and cut into small chunks

- One cup of Coconut Milk

- Half teaspoon of Salt

- One and a half teaspoons of Fresh Ginger grated, peeled

Required Equipment:

- Food Processor or Immersion Blender

Directions

1. Firstly, add the potatoes to a clean stockpot filled with water. Then bring to a boil over high heat approximately fifteen minutes or until it is fork tender.

2. As soon as the potatoes are finished, drain the water. In the same pot, add the chicken broth, ginger and salt.

3. Next blend the potatoes until smooth with an immersion blender. Serve hot to enjoy.

One Pan Garlic & Herb Chicken Drumsticks with Patty Pan Squash

Preparation Time: 5 Minutes

Cook Time: 35 Minutes

Total Time: 40 Minutes

Calories: 360kcal

Yields: 3 Servings

Recipes:

- Two tablespoons of ghee

- One pound of chicken drumsticks can sub chicken thighs or breasts

- 1/3 cup of fresh oregano, chopped

- Two cloves of garlic, minced

- Two teaspoons of fresh sage, minced

- Two teaspoons of fresh thyme, minced

- Salt to taste

- Three to five cups of patty pan squash, ends trimmed and quartered

- Pepper to taste

Directions

1. Oven to 400 degrees Fahrenheit.

2. Next heat a large clean oven-safe, non-stick skillet over medium to high heat.

3. Next Add ghee to the pan. As soon as the ghee has melted add garlic and then sauté for one minute.

4. Next add the chicken drumsticks to the pan and then sear for three to four minutes or until it

appears golden. Flip and then cook for additional two to three minutes.

5. Next add in pepper, chopped herbs and salt.

6. Next place pan in the oven & bake for twenty to twenty-five minutes. Add in the squash. Toss and then place back into the oven for additional ten minutes or until the chicken is cooked through att internal temperature of 165 degrees Fahrenheit.

7. Serve to enjoy.

One-Pan Chicken Bake

Preparation Time: 10 Minutes

Cook Time: 40 Minutes

Total Time: 50 Minutes

Yields: 4 Servings

Recipes:

- One tablespoon of avocado oil or ghee

- One pound of chicken thighs (skin on or off, bone in-or boneless)

- One teaspoon of garlic powder

- One teaspoon of dried oregano

- Two tablespoons of capers

- One teaspoon of onion powder

- Half medium yellow onion, sliced

- Three cups of diced parsnips (about one large or two small)

- One cup of kalamata olives, drained

- ¼ cup of parsley, chopped

- Half lemon, sliced

Directions

1. Oven to 425 degrees Fahrenheit.

2. Place an ovenproof large clean cast iron skillet and warm it up over medium heat with one tablespoon of avocado oil for about one to two minutes. Using paper towels, pat dry the chicken and then season all sides with pepper and a pinch of salt.

3. As soon as the skillet is hot, add the chicken with the skin-side down.

4. Next cook the chicken for about six to eight minutes, until the chicken is just browned.

5. Next as the chicken is cooking, combine the garlic, oregano, the sea salt left, onion and pepper in a clean small container.

6. As soon as the chicken is done, flip and then cook for around one minute, then add the parsnips, sliced onions, capers and olives to the pan. Season all by sprinkling the spice blend over the entire skillet.

7. Next add in the lemon slices around the pan and then place the skillet in the oven. Roast for approximately twenty-five minutes, until the chicken is well cooked through.

8. Serve to enjoy, garnish with fresh chopped parsley.

Chicken Saltimbocca

Preparation Time: 5 Minutes

Cook Time: 25 Minutes

Total Time: 30 Minutes

Yields: 4 Servings

Recipes:

- One tablespoon of ghee or coconut oil, divided

- One pound of chicken thighs

- One teaspoon of minced garlic

- Half yellow onions, sliced

- Prosciutto - one slice for each piece of chicken

- Half cup of chicken broth

- Six fresh sage leaves

- juice and zest of half lemon

- Pepper, to taste

- Salt, to taste

Directions

1. Firstly, season the chicken with salt & pepper. Place one to two large sage leaves on each piece, and half a slice of the prosciutto on top.

2. Next heat a large cast-iron skillet over medium to high heat with ghee. Swirl the pan to coat. Add chicken; cook six to seven minutes per side.

3. Take out the chicken from pan and reserve warm.

4. Next add the ghee left to the pan. Sauté the garlic until it fragrant, around thirty seconds. Add onions, chicken broth, lemon juice and zest to the pan. Crank heat to high and decrease sauce down until it thickens much and flavours, around seven to ten minutes.

5. Next about halfway through the cooking time, add the prosciutto left. Pay attention to the sauce, it can go from watery to dry very rapidly.

6. Lower the heat to a simmer as soon as it thickens up. Add take the chicken back to the pan to warm it and then coat with the sauce.

7. You can spoon more sauce over the chicken.

8. If preferred, drizzle in balsamic vinegar on top to enjoy.

Cauliflower Tabouli and Salmon

Meal Prep

Preparation Time: 20 Minutes

Cook Time: 10 Minutes

Total Time: 30 Minutes

Calories: 510kcal

Yields: 4 Servings

Recipes:

- One medium head cauliflower riced

- Four 4-ounce pieces wild caught sockeye salmon

- Two green onions, thinly sliced

- Half bunch of flat leaf parsley, chopped

- 2/3 cup of English cucumber, diced

- One large Lemon zest and juice

- 1/4 cup of olive oil

- 2/3 cup of roma tomato diced, seeds and core removed

- Two tablespoons of avocado oil

- Half teaspoon of Sea Salt

- Two cloves of garlic, minced

Optional

- Lemon slices for garnish

- Fresh mint

Directions

1. Oven to 400 degrees Fahrenheit. Carefully line a baking sheet with clean foil greased with one tablespoon of avocado oil.

2. Next place the salmon fillets with the skin side down onto the baking sheet; drizzle the avocado oil left over salmon and then season with 1/4 teaspoon of salt. Put in the middle of the oven & bake for seven to ten minutes, or until it is firm, flakes and opaque.

3. As the salmon bakes, combine recipes left in a large clean mixing bowl/container until well incorporated. Put aside.

4. As soon as it is cooked, serve salmon along with cauliflower tabouli.

5. Enjoy!

Tilapia Lettuce Wraps with Mango Papaya Salsa

Preparation Time: 30 Minutes

Cook Time: 5 Minutes

Total Time: 35 Minutes

Calories: 311kcal

Yields; 2 Servings

Recipes:

For the Mango Papaya Salsa:

- 1/4 Papaya diced (around one cup)

- One Mango diced (around one cup)

- Two tablespoons of Fresh Cilantro chopped

- One Shallot minced

- Salt to taste

- Two tablespoons of Fresh Lime Juice White Vinegar
  would be an ok substitute

For the Fish:

- One teaspoon of Garlic Powder

- Half teaspoon of Salt

- One teaspoon of Dried Oregano

- One teaspoon of Flour Cassava Flour

- Two tablespoons of Lard Ghee, Coconut Oil or
  Avocado Oil are fine as well

- One to One and a half pounds Tilapia fresh or
  thawed if frozen

For Serving:

- Two Radishes thinly sliced

- One Head Butter Lettuce cleaned and separated

Directions

1. Combine all salsa recipes and then add salt to taste, put aside.

2. Combine all the dry recipes for the fish in a clean small container and then stir well to combine.

3. Now sprinkle the mixture over all sides of the fish.

4. Also, you should rub the mixture into the fish, ensure the entire fish is seasoned.

5. Add the lard (or other oil) into a large clean frying pan.

6. As soon as pan is hot and lard is melted, gently lay fish fillets in the pan and cook for two minutes per side or until the fish gets flakey.

7. Next place fish into lettuce leaves, lay radish slices on top and then add salsa. Serve straightaway to enjoy.

Turkey and Mushroom Lettuce Wrap

Preparation Time: 30 Minutes

Cook Time: 15 Minutes

Total Time: 45 Minutes

Calories: 493kcal

Yields: 4 Servings

Recipes:

- Extra Virgin Olive Oil

- One and a half to two pounds Ground Turkey

- Four Green Onions, thinly sliced

- Three cloves of garlic, minced

- Eight ounces of can Sliced Water Chestnuts, drained and coarsely chopped

- One pound of Button Mushrooms chopped

- One tablespoon of Fish Sauce Two tablespoons if omitting wine

- One tablespoon of White Vinegar

- Twelve Butter Lettuce leaves one to two heads of lettuce

- One bunch Cilantro leaves chopped

Directions

1. Heat one tablespoon of olive oil in a large clean sauté pan over medium to high heat.

2. Now add the turkey and cook until lightly browned, around three to five minutes, ensure you crumble the turkey as it cooks.

3. Take out the turkey from the pan, add one more tablespoon of olive oil and then add garlic and onions to the pan.

4. Cook until appears translucent, approximately thirty seconds to one minute.

5. Now add the rice vinegar, mushrooms, fish sauce and wine.

6. Now cook for additional three to five minutes, occasionally stirring.

7. Finally, add the ground meat and water chestnuts back into the pan, and then allow it cook for some minutes until the liquid has decreased.

8. Now stir in cilantro then season with pepper and salt, to taste.

9. To serve, put some tablespoons of the beef mixture into the middle of a lettuce leaf, taco-style.

Roasted Squash, Beef and Arugula Salad

Preparation Time: 10 Minutes

Cook Time: 20 Minutes

Total Time: 30 Minutes

Calories: 394kcal

Yields: 4 Servings

Recipes:

- Extra Virgin Olive Oil
- Two Delicata Squash halved, cleaned & sliced into half-inch slices
- One pound of Ground Beef
- Salt

- One teaspoon of Italian Seasonings

- One teaspoon of Garlic Powder

- One Onion chopped

- Two tablespoons of White Wine Vinegar

- Seven ounces of Arugula

Directions

1. Oven to 450 degrees Fahrenheit.

2. Now place the squash on a clean baking sheet with about two tablespoons of olive oil and half teaspoon of salt.

3. Next toss and then place the squash in a layer on the baking sheet.

4. Next bake the squash for around twenty minutes or until the squash is fork tender and begins to brown.

5. As the squash is cooking, begin cooking the ground meat.

6. In a clean sauté pan, add garlic powder, the ground beef, half teaspoon of salt and Italian seasonings.

7. Ensure to break up the meat as you are cooking at high heat for approximately three to five minutes or until browned.

8. With a clean slotted spoon remove the ground beef from the pan and then place on a different plate.

9. Add the onion to the pan and then sauté over medium to heat until it appears translucent, about three to five minutes.

10.   As soon as the onion has finished cooking, use a slotted spoon to take them out from the pan & add them to the beef.

For the Salad:

1. Firstly, toss the arugula with the vinegar.

2. Next add the ground beef mixture to the arugula &

then layer the squash on top.

3. Add vinegar and salt to taste.

Pulled Pork Stuffed Squash

Preparation Time: 1 Minute

Cook Time: 30 Minutes

Total Time: 31 Minutes

Yields: 2 Servings

Recipes:

- Two servings leftover pulled pork
- One delicata squash, seeds removed and cut in halves

To Serve:

- Sea salt
- Avocado Slices

Directions

1. Oven to 400 degrees Fahrenheit. Carefully line a baking sheet with clean parchment paper.

2. Next place the squash face down on the baking sheet lined with parchment paper and then bake for thirty minutes or until it is golden brown and forkable.

3. When the squash has around 10 minutes to complete, heat a clean medium-sized skillet over medium heat for two minutes.

4. Next place the leftover pork in the pan. If necessary, break up using a clean wooden spoon. Let it crisp on all sides for around five to six minutes. Brown the pork on a side for some minutes without turning it, then flip it for the other side until it is browned.

5. Next carefully take out the squash from the oven, flip over, and stuff with pork.

6. Next top with sea salt and avocado slices, if wanted.

7. Enjoy!

Cauliflower Rice Salmon Poke Bowl Meal Prep

Preparation Time: 20 Minutes

Total Time: 20 Minutes

Calories: 334kcal

Yields: 4 Servings

Recipes:

- One head of cauliflower, grated

- One teaspoon of avocado oil

- Two Carrots, shredded

- Sixteen ounces wild caught salmon

- One tablespoon of rice vinegar

- One medium Avocado, thinly sliced

- Sesame Seeds for serving, optional

- One green onion, thinly sliced

Directions

1. Firstly, place cauliflower rice on the stovetop cook over medium heat in a bit of avocado oil for eight to ten minutes, until it is softened and lightly browned. Put aside.

2. Next cube the salmon into small chunks and then season with a splash of rice vinegar and little Himalayan sea salt.

3. Rinse and chop all the avocado veggies.

To Assemble:

Share the cauliflower rice between bowls and top with avocado, sliced veggies, raw salmon, white sesame seeds, a splash more of rice vinegar and green onion. Store in the fridge for four days.

Turmeric Ginger Salmon in Foil

Meal Prep

Preparation Time: 10 Minutes

Cook Time: 30 Minutes

Total Time: 40 Minutes

Calories: 426kcal

Yields: 3 Servings

Recipes:

- Two medium sweet potatoes sliced in half lengthwise

- Three 4-ounce of salmon filets

- Five ounces of broccoli florets

- One and a half teaspoons of turmeric

- One teaspoon of Ground Ginger

- Four tablespoons of oil

Directions

1. Oven to 375 degrees Fahrenheit.

2. Next place the sliced sweet potatoes on a large clean baking sheet.

3. Next spoon one tablespoon of the oil over the salmon filets. Sprinkle with half teaspoon of turmeric.

4. Next place the sweet potatoes into the oven and then bake at 375 degrees Fahrenheit for thirty minutes.

5. Next place the three salmon filets in the middle of three large squares of foil.

6. Share the broccoli among the three packs around the salmon.

7. Next in a ramekin, mix together ginger, the oil left and turmeric.

8. With a clean pastry brush, coat the broccoli and salmon with the oil.

9. Next carefully wrap the ends of the foil closed and then place gently on a baking sheet.

10. Now bake at 375 degrees Fahrenheit for the twenty minutes left with the sweet potatoes.

11. Take out of the oven and share into three meal prep bowl/containers.

Sheet Pan Steak Dinner

Preparation Time: 20 Minutes

Cook Time: 30 Minutes

Total Time: 50 Minutes

Yields: 4 Servings

Recipes:

- Salt

- Four to five Sweet Potatoes, peeled and chopped

- Two pints White Mushrooms, sliced

- Extra Virgin Olive Oil

- Two pounds of Flank Steak

- Italian Seasonings

Directions

1. Oven to 450 degrees Fahrenheit.

2. Next toss potatoes with one tablespoon olive oil, half teaspoon of salt and one teaspoon Italian seasonings.

3. Next pour on the sweet potatoes on a clean sheet pan.

4. Next place into the oven for twenty minutes.

5. Meanwhile, toss the mushrooms, in the same bowl that held the half teaspoon of Italian seasonings, sweet potatoes and 1/4 teaspoon of salt.

6. Generously season all sides of the steak with salt. one teaspoon of Italian Seasonings and also a few tablespoons of olive oil.

7. Take out the pan from the oven and then move the sweet potatoes to one side of the baking sheet to make space for the steak and mushrooms.

8. Next add the steak and mushrooms to the pan.

9. Next put back the pan into the oven and cook for an extra fifteen minutes.

10.   Next broil for two to four minutes or until the top of the steak is slightly brown.

11. Take out the pan from the oven.

12. Allow the meat sit for ten minutes.

13. As the meat is sitting, toss the potatoes and mushrooms.

14. Next slice the meat

15. Serve to enjoy.

Conclusion

The cellular connections of the intestinal wall become disrupted in leaky gut syndrome, allowing undigested food and germs to "leak" into the circulation. Many autoimmune illnesses, such as IBS and celiac disease, have been linked to a leaky gut. However, it is not yet a well-known medical illness, and more research is needed to figure out what causes it and how to treat it properly.

Although the cause of the leaky gut syndrome is unknown, there is evidence that following a "leaky gut diet" can help relieve symptoms. Gluten, dairy, sugar, and other typical irritants should be avoided, focusing on healthy fats, fermented foods, probiotic supplements, and lifestyle factors.

Eat foods that encourage the growth of healthy gut bacteria, such as fruits, cultured dairy products, healthy fats, lean meats, and fibre and fermented vegetables, to help prevent leaky gut.

The recipes in this book are adequate for all cooking skill levels.

Enjoy!